ASPERGERS SYNDROME

A Complete Aspergers Syndrome Cure Guide

(A Complete Guide to Understanding, Loving, and Communicating)

Julius Mejia

Published by Tomas Edwards

© **Julius Mejia**

All Rights Reserved

Aspergers Syndrome: A Complete Aspergers Syndrome Cure Guide (A Complete Guide to Understanding, Loving, and Communicating)

ISBN 978-1-990268-71-7

All rights reserved. No part of this guide may be reproduced in any form without permission in writing from the publisher except in the case of brief quotations embodied in critical articles or reviews.

Legal & Disclaimer

The information contained in this book is not designed to replace or take the place of any form of medicine or professional medical advice. The information in this book has been provided for educational and entertainment purposes only.

The information contained in this book has been compiled from sources deemed reliable, and it is accurate to the best of the Author's knowledge; however, the Author cannot guarantee its accuracy and validity and cannot be held liable for any errors or omissions. Changes are periodically made to this book. You must consult your doctor or get professional medical advice before using any of the suggested remedies, techniques, or information in this book.

Upon using the information contained in this book, you agree to hold harmless the Author from and against any damages, costs, and expenses, including any legal fees potentially resulting from the application of any of the information provided by this guide. This disclaimer applies to any damages or injury caused by the use and application, whether directly or indirectly, of any advice or information presented, whether for breach of contract, tort, negligence, personal injury, criminal intent, or under any other cause of action.

You agree to accept all risks of using the information presented inside this book. You need to consult a professional medical practitioner in order to ensure you are both able and healthy enough to participate in this program.

Table of Contents

INTRODUCTION 1

CHAPTER 1: ASPERGER'S SYNDROME 5

CHAPTER 2: TREATMENTS FOR ASPERGER SYNDROME ... 25

CHAPTER 3: CHARACTERISTICS OF ASPERGER SYNDROME 44

CHAPTER 4: "ASPER -- WHAT?" 54

CHAPTER 5: OVERVIEW OF THE ASPERGER SYNDROME .. 70

CHAPTER 6: ASPERGERS SYNDROME TREATMENTS, THERAPIES AND MEDICATION. 98

CONCLUSION 124

Introduction

There is a huge gap between the reality of this condition and what the masses have been fed, which has made Asperger's a very mysterious and misunderstood condition for many years. This book attempts to clear the dust and educate open-minded readers into this condition.

Most people with Asperger's syndrome are intelligent and they usually possess an average to above-average intelligence. Cognitive ability is not affected by this condition. One way to assist and guide a person with this condition is to be patient and to establish rapport. Although maintaining a relationship is quite difficult for some people diagnosed with Asperger's syndrome, the hopeful assertion is that communicative and social abilities are skills and can, therefore, be learned.

Nowadays, different and new medical conditions are being discovered. But, this book is not a research journal review. This book was created with the belief that the general population be accurately informed of Asperger's Disorder before imposing any customs that we may perceive as "normal." People need to know the potential causes, symptoms, and various treatments, how can it affect the lives of the affected people, and the importance of support groups.

However, there are some people who are not willing to learn. The approach depends on family, friends, teachers, or and health care providers. Learning about the largely misrepresented, which include Asperger's, has the potential to reignite the essence of connection through empathy and understanding.

This book will be beneficial for you if:

• You know someone who has been diagnosed with Asperger's Syndrome and you want to know how you can help and assist them

• You want to learn about this condition to share knowledge to other people

• You want to know more about this syndrome and you want to expand your thoughts and ideas about it

Asperger's Syndrome is also known as "having a dash of autism". However, although it has been said that this is the mildest form of autism, the person diagnosed with this condition processes the world differently from a normal functioning brain and will, thus, exhibit a range of distinct behaviors. This syndrome needs to be shared and discussed for us to better understand and effectively support people in this situation.

Thanks again for downloading this book. I hope you find much value in it.

Chapter 1: Asperger's Syndrome

Asperger syndrome (AS), is also called Asperger disorder (AD) or just Asperger. It is a condition which belongs to autism spectrum disorder or (ASD). The patient suffering from this condition experiences challenges in social interaction and more so nonverbal communication. The child or patient will have repetitive and also restricted patterns of behavior and also interests. Though it belongs to the broad autism disorder, there exists a major difference by its relative conservation of linguistic and cognitive growth. The person will have clumsy tendencies and a haltingly use of language. In 2013, Asperger's diagnosis was removed from the Diagnostic and Statistical Manual of Mental Disorders (DSM-5). But it was later replaced with an autism diagnosis on an excessive scale.

It bears a its name from the Han's Asperger's, the Austrian pediatrician who studied it in 1944 and explained that the children who he met during his practice were deficient in nonverbal communication skills while at the same time demonstrated minimal empathy when they were among their peers. He also noted that these children were clumsy in their physical interactions. But in 1981, Asperger's syndrome modern concept was born and it went through seasons of popularization and became the standardized diagnosis 1990s. It is a condition that abounds with controversy and many unanswered questions.

Asperger's real cause has remained a mystery till today. Although research has fronted many suggestions like the likelihood of a genetic basis, but even then, the genetic cause remains unknown while medical advancement like the famed brain imaging methodologies have not been specific in identifying clear and concise pathology. On treatment there has not found one single treatment and the interventions that are there and their impact on treating the condition have been enhanced but scanty data. The intervention of this disease is geared towards the improvement of it symptoms and the functions. The bedrock of the treatment of Asperger's is the behavioral therapy which focuses on certain deficits in order to buttonhole poor communication skills and the obsessive and repetitive routines in this people or children and finally address the physical clumsiness. Many children will have their situation improve as they grow old into adulthood. But even when they are old one will still notice communication and social difficulties. Researchers and many people with this condition have advocated a change in attitude and come to agree with the view that difference occurring are not a disability but a condition which can treat.

Motor and Sensory Perception

Individuals who suffer from Asperger syndrome may exhibit symptoms that stand alone and are contrary to the diagnosis. But they also affect not only the individual but also the family. The major differences include challenges with their motor skills, emotions, sleep and their perception.

People who suffer from Asperger's have wonderful visual perception and near-perfect auditory reception. Children with this condition always portray great perception of small changes particularly in patterns and arrangements of objects which are called well-known images. It is an area that acts as a domain- to these children and involves the processing of detailed characteristics. Conversely, when compared to people with high-functioning autism, people with AS have shortfalls in tasks which involve visual-spatial perception, visual memory and auditory perception.

Reports from people who suffer from Asperger's and ASD give evidence of their unusual sensory and at times perceptual skills and feelings. At times they are also highly sensitive or at times insensitive to light, sound and other stimuli. These sensory reactions are found in different developmental disorders and are not particular people suffering from AS or ASD. But there is more evidence of decreased responsiveness to sensory stimuli, although several studies show no differences.

THE OUTLOOK FOR PEOPLE WITH ASPERGER'S SYNDROME

Asperger's Syndrome is a condition that puts the children's and adults at risk where they can develop other and serious conditions which could include ADHD, depression, schizophrenia, and serious obsessive-compulsive disorders. Research has also help improve treatment options for this condition and they are readily available for people suffering from Asperger's Syndrome.

One advantage with people suffering from this is that the degree of intelligence is said to be higher than the average or a little higher than average, Asperger's syndrome patients are able to run their day to day roles without facing many challenges. These patients may be destined how ever to live with their inability to socialize well with their friends and workmates through adulthood.

Can Asperger's Syndrome Be Prevented?

The greatest question has been whether Asperger's syndrome can be cured. But it has been discovered that early diagnosis and enhanced treatment can help improve and amend the functioning and the quality of life.

Securing Services

Many people have found themselves in a dilemma after discovering that their child is sick with Asperger's Syndrome. After visiting the hospital and ascertaining the condition of the child, it is recommended that one starts by making contacts with the local authorities to find where organizations that cater for people with this condition area found. It is also important to get acquainted with his child's educational rights. In many nations who have realized the need to cater for children with this condition, the law states that public schools set aside educational services for people of ages three to twenty one who have disabilities which includes Asperger's. Also, there may be state and local laws or policies to aid children with Asperger's.

Since it the treatment of Asperger's a joint affair between the parents, minders and members of the medical profession, it is vital for the school personnel to key out objectives and establishes a specialized and individualized education program (IEP). These programs or IEPs are tailored to fit the child suffering from Asperger's Syndrome's specific needs that are based on the evaluation of her level of disability.

What School Programs Entail

It is of paramount importance that the parent asses the type of services that are available in t he school where his taking child. It is important to have a checklist based on informed decision. Therefore there are important qualities that one has to look for.

The school should have working groups. These groups should be small in size so as to give maximum attention to the child or individual suffering from Asperger's Syndrome. The program will do the child or adult an injustice if it does not have a communication specialist. The role of this specialist is to train the child in social skills so as enhance his chances of coordinating with his friends and family members without causing problems. It is therefore important for the communication specialist to have a great interest or a calling into this kind of work. It is quite involving and calls for a person who is endowed with lots of patience.

A parent should also have a keen eye when he visits such an institution seeking a placement for his child. She should look for a structured setting that creates room for a social interaction among the children who are suffering from Asperger's Syndrome. If the settings are not good enough particularly when it comes to the size of space for these children, then the children may suffer stress instead of improving on their health state. One should also be keen on the supervision levels in such institutions. Since most of these children are very anti-social in their interaction with the rest, then poor supervision may lead them into harming one another. The parameters that a parent should check should include the teaching staff in this school. The parent should be concerned if the teacher cannot impact real-life skills. It should be the paramount reason that such an institution or school was opened. The teachers should be in the forefront of noting the child's special talents and interests. The teacher should go further and impact them on the child to make the program very effective.

The checklist should not end until the teacher can show and demonstrate a desire to individualize and internalize the curriculum. If the school does not have a sensitive and compassionate counselor, then the school does not meet the criteria of good school for child suffering from Asperger's Syndrome. These children require emotional attachment and well being. So the counselor serves liaison or the go-between with the family of the child. Asperger's Syndrome is a condition that is no respecter of status quo or nationalities. Therefore it is paramount for such schools to put much emphasis on diversity, empathy and compassion for these students.

It is therefore important for the parent to keep abreast of the news as far as the programs in these institutions are concerned. The classroom environment where one's child is schooling should be put into perspective. Without constant communication between the teacher and the parent will go a long way in monitoring the progress of the child? It is therefore advisable to have a diary that oscillates between the teacher and the parent so as not to have a lapse in communication that could be detrimental in the child's treatment program.

Treatment Strategies

Asperger's treatment is arranged towards the improvement of communication, behavior management and he child's social skills. Therefore there is always a need where this treatment program can be adjusted based on the need of the child. What other advice can a parent be given? He should try as much as possible to make use of his child's strong points and be at the forefront of encouraging her to dig into what interests him in school and also at home. It also recommended that there be groups that are action-oriented and which are focused on counseling the child which can be very helpful.

Asperger's Syndrome - Home Treatment

The role of taking care of a child with Asperger's Syndrome should not end with the medics and other professionals. It also calls for the parent getting to know about the condition and applying the skills for the child at home. It will help ease the pressure on the parents when they are without the medics at home. It will also create an active role for the parent and ease the stress that comes with counting one's losses. And since there are programs for taking care of these children at home, then a parent should study and apply them. The love and the experience that a parent receives in a supportive role go a long way in improving the well-being of this child. It demystifies the notion that this child with Asperger's Syndrome is not an only child. One will get to know that this child is a child like any other who has weaknesses and strengths and requires patience, support and proper understanding to improve their lives.

The benefits of one getting acquainted with this condition by educating yourself brings with it great change. You will be able to set goals of what you want to achieve with your child on the treatment of Asperger's Syndrome. One will get to know that the following objectives are achievable. They include your child's developing independence while at the same time help the child succeed at home and in school. So where can the parent get information on Asperger's syndrome and learn on how to handle his child? One avenue is by consulting a doctor and by also making contacts with Asperger's organizations. When you have acquired vital information about Asperger's Syndrome as a parent will in the reduction of stress among your family members' and experience your child succeed.

General Strategies for Success

In summary, there are the tips that a parent and the groups minding a child with Asperger's syndrome should have. These ideas may apply to one child while they may not work for others. It is therefore paramount for a parent to be creative and very flexible in exercising these strategies. Another vital tool is to have a willingness to learn about Asperger's Syndrome from the doctor or reliable sources to help you in raising your child with minimal stress.

Children who suffer from Asperger's syndrome are able to benefit from routes that are formed in them on a daily basis. These daily routines apply when it comes to meal times, when they are involved in their homework and when they go to bed. It is worth noting that these are planned as specific rules which should be consistent with milestones of achievable expectations which will mean little stress and untold confusion for these children. Many children and adults with Asperger's syndrome are readily reachable when it comes to communication through verbal assignments and training. They find it a bit hard when it comes to nonverbal assignments and teaching. It is therefore very important to have concise, direct, mode of training. These programs have been developed and one can get them from Asperger's Syndrome organizations that have been on a mission to help children with these problems.

Children and adults with Asperger's syndrome are always faced with the challenges of grasping the "big picture". Due to the challenges that they go through, they tend to visualize things as a part and not able to see it as a whole object. With this kind of understanding, then the teaching program should be made in "parts-to-whole-teaching-methodology. It is an approach that should start with section of a concept with more additions to it to establish encompassing ideas.

Like we have seen earlier, these children are good on the practical side of training than on the theoretical one. A teacher should therefore try as much as possible to visual supports which include schedules and written materials that aid with the organizational of the child which counts a lot in the well being of the child. Children suffering from Asperger's Syndrome are very sensitive to little, little changes. The teacher should try s much as possible to remove any thing that can cause background noises. A serious destruction to these children is when a clock is ticking. It destructs them and it may take time before they can come back and concentrate on their programs. Even the humming of a fluorescent light may be enough to distract a child suffering from Asperger's Syndrome.

Other children who could be suffering from autism spectrum disorders which also includes Asperger's syndrome have a high affinity for video games. They are also fascinated by computers and screen-based media like a TV. To safeguard the wellbeing of your child it is advisable to keep televisions, computers and video games from your child's bedroom. Spending much time watching television or playing video games by this child will take away the number of hours he should sleep. Having enough sleep is a medical advice for children suffering from Asperger's Syndrome. If this child is not able to get enough sleep, then her ASD symptoms may move from worse to worst.

Children who suffer from Asperger's syndrome take a lot of time to grow to maturity. It is important for parents to know that and therefore the expectation for them to behave according to their age should not be there. So it will be absurd to expect them to behave their age.

One area that hampers quick treatment in children and people who suffer from Asperger's Syndrome is stress. For a parent, it is important to look for what triggers stress in your child and remove them. The training in these children should be based on preparing this child for challenges of life. It is a parent's responsibility to train them on how to cope with these challenges of life. Life will not always be smooth and dependable on a second person. It therefore calls for a parent preparing the child to cope with new situations and challenges.

Chapter 2: Treatments For Asperger Syndrome

Asperger syndrome is not a disease and there is no exact cure for this syndrome. However, you can prevent the affect of this syndrome in your child by some treatment and learning programs. Asperger syndrome is very hard to treat because the symptoms of this disease may vary depending on the nature of an individual, his or her age, his surrounding environment, his social environment, and many more. We have to consider these concepts before proceeding our treatment. An Asperger child may face conundrums in the initial phase of his life but if the parents and teachers provide him necessary guidance and training, then he or she can come over the affects of

Asperger syndrome and live a normal life with this syndrome.

Asperger children generally face problems in their middle school and high school life because they have quite different behaviour as compared to their peers. But when they become adult, they can learn how to cope with this syndrome and its symptoms and live a normal life. So providing necessary guidance and training is necessary for these children. Here are some of the treatments for Asperger syndrome: --

Applied Behaviour Analysis

Applied Behaviour Analysis (ABA) is the use of various behaviour analysis methods that were adopted through the analysis and research in this field. ABA is not a single treatment approach but a combination of various different approaches to train an Asperger child how to cope with his or her symptoms. ABA is often difficult to understand until you see it in action. There are various methods of ABA as described below: --

An antecedent

Antecedent is the verbal or physical stimulus like command or request. Asperger syndrome child often face problems to understand the basic context in which a sentence is used like they have problem to understand whether 'Please pick that book' is a command or a request or some other kind of sentence. This may come from the environment or from another person.

Resulting Behaviour

Resulting behaviour is the way in which an Asperger child responds to certain kind of sentence. It is the response or lack of response to the antecedent described earlier.

A consequence

Consequence depends on the behaviour of Asperger child and includes positive reinforcement of the desired behaviour or no reaction.

ABA works in the most common way our brain works i.e. rewarding a child every time when he or she achieves a certain milestone in learning. A human brain has a rewarding technique in which it generates reward hormones like dopamine whenever the person achieves something personally or mentally in his life. This rewarding technique motivates a human being to learn new concepts in his life. In ABA, a child is provided with many different skill sets depending on his personal behaviour and the level of his Asperger syndrome. The child is provided with repeated opportunities to learn and practice each skill in a variety of settings. Each time a child achieves desired result, he or she receives positive reinforcement like a verbal praise or something highly motivating for them like a small piece of candy.

Verbal Behaviour

Verbal behaviour is used to teach proper communication skills and using the principles of ABA and some of the theories of famous behaviourist B. F. Skinner. Asperger syndrome children have a different perception to the language as compared to normal children and that's why Verbal Behaviour therapy plays an important role to teach how to teach language to them. As I have explained in my book earlier that these children face difficulties in learning the abstract concepts of language like metaphors, parables, phrases, irony, sarcasm, and idioms. This is the reason why some behaviourists have developed Verbal Behaviour to teach language to Asperger syndrome child. In Verbal Behaviour, a student learns how words can help obtain desired results or objects. Verbal Behaviour therapy avoids focusing on words as mere labels. This therapy focuses on four word types as follows: --

Mand: -- A request, such as "Cookie," to ask for a Cookie.

Tact: -- A comment used to share an experience or draw someone's attention, such as "airplane" to point out an airplane.

Intraverbal: -- A word used to either answer a question or respond, such as "Where are you going?" "To school."

Echoic: -- A repeated or echoed word, such as "Cookie!" "Cookie?"

In the most basic form of learning Verbal Behaviour therapy, a child learns how to use mands in the most basic form of language. For example the child with Asperger learns that saying a single word "Cookie" can simply produce Cookie. This notion goes deep inside their brain as a most common form of word and he receives a reward by his brain when next time he repeats this word. Immediately after the child makes a request, the therapist reinforces the lesson by repeating the word and presenting the requested item. Then, the therapist again uses the same word in same or similar context. This way a child really learns the common difference between various words and sentences and his brain saves them accordingly in his brain.

Pivotal Response Treatment

Pivotal Response Treatment (PRT) is another widely used form of behavioural intervention used to treat Asperger child that was developed by Dr. Robert L. Koegel, Dr. Laura Shreibman, and Dr. Lynn Kenn Koegel at the University or California.

PRT is the set of best studied and validated behavioural form of treatment for Asperger syndrome. PRT is basically derived from ABA and it is play based and child initiated. The therapist used a direct approach of targeting the pivotal areas of a child's development rather than targeting individual behaviour in PRT. Some common emphasis in PRT is motivation, response to cues, self-management and the initiation of social interactions. By targeting these critical areas, a therapist tries to produce broad improvements across other areas of sociability, academic skills, communication and behaviour.

Motivation strategy is an important of PRT approach. It emphasize on the natural reinforcement e.g. if a child makes meaningful attempt to request like a stuffed animal, the reward is the stuffed animal and not a candy or other unrelated reward. This way a child makes a direct connection of his reward with the request he made and it helps him to learn the precise meaning of a request made. PRT needs the participation of every person involved in the child's life like his father, mother, brother, sister, or any other relative. PRT describes how to adopt a lifestyle by the family of child so that he or she learns some basic skills on the go.

Cognitive Behaviour Therapy

Cognitive Behaviour Therapy (CBT) is used to help a child with Asperger syndrome to regulate his emotions, develop impulse control, and improve their behaviour as a positive result. CBT is an effective therapy that helps a child to understand his or her thoughts and feelings more precisely so that they can learn how to respond to them in a more effective way. As I have described earlier in my book, a child having Asperger syndrome doesn't consciously know the reason of his behaviour and attitude towards his surrounding atmosphere and society. He or she feels very annoyed sometimes because his mind doesn't probably behave according to his thoughts and emotions. CBT is a best therapy to teach a child how to control his emotions and thoughts in a more precise way rather than just acting weird in some emotional conditions.

Cognition is most important to justify a person's thought process and emotions. A normal person knows how to react to different situations he faces in a day to day life. But a Asperger child is not able to relate the circumstances to his thoughts and emotions and often act in a weird way in some conditions. CBT has proved to help in reducing anxious and depressed feelings inside an Asperger child. CBT tends to make some changes in thoughts and perception through a change in cognition. Therapists proved to reduce challenging behaviours among Asperger children using CBT such as interruptions, meltdowns or angry outbursts, obsessions, aggression, and shouting in many cases.

CBT is most effective for the treatment of Asperger syndrome because it can be individualized to a patient, depending on his cognitive behaviour, thought process, and emotional stress level. It is very effective at improving very specific behaviours and challenges in each child or an adult.

Occupational Therapy

Another commonly used therapy for Asperger syndrome is Occupational Therapy (OT). OT addresses a combination of cognitive, physical, and motor skills for the treatment of Asperger among children. Its main motivation is to help a child to gain age-relevant independence and participate more fully and functionally in life. OT consist combination of many skills for including appropriate play or leisure skills, learning and self-care skills.

A person related to a certain age has different approach and motivation towards his life. A child would give preference to game rather than learning, whereas an adult would like to indulge himself in learning skills rather to play games. But an Asperger syndrome child would act quite weirdly in some cases and he would love to indulge himself in learning skills and that too in a very precise extent. He would love to learn certain subject and put his maximum concentration on it. But he should not learn other subjects in this condition and his school grade will fall. In OT, therapists teach the children how to put their concentration on each and every aspect of their life to bring forward a real identity of them.

Physical Therapy

Many children and adults suffering from Asperger syndrome face challenges to control their normal body functioning with motor skills such as sitting, walking, jumping, and running. Physical Therapy (PT) is used to focus on problems with movement that cause limitations in normal functioning of an Asperger syndrome child. Many children suffering from Asperger have to face difficulties in learning most common physical activities like writing. This put a halt in the functioning of their normal life and they become depressed and anxious.

Certified physical therapists employ various strategies to deliver physical therapy to these children with an evaluation of their abilities and development level. Therapy sessions usually run for half hour to an hour, including assisted movements, various forms of exercise and use of orthopaedic equipments.

One of the great physical therapy that is becoming famous for the treatment of Asperger syndrome nowadays is Aikido. Aikido is a form of martial arts technique that emphasises on the self defence of a person without seriously hurting his opponent. Researchers have found that the child suffering from Asperger syndrome often finds it difficult to play some sports that includes the involvement of more than one player like that traditional basketball or soccer game. This is the main reason why these children don't get an opportunity to develop certain parts of their brain for developing motor skills.

Aikido is a marital art form that depends only on the movement of two partners. An Asperger child generally has a single focus and by placing the child in a situation where he or she only has to deal with one partner, odds of success increase to a great extent. We know that success in any sport is related to motor co-ordination. Many Asperger syndrome kids have a deficit motor co-ordinating condition and they have to face many challenges in participating in team sports. Researchers have discovered that these children often find it difficult in tossing and catching a ball, hopping, or following the directions related to their physical movements. Now, because Aikido develops whole body integration, eye-hand co-ordination becomes unnecessary.

Since most Aikido techniques involve both throwing and falling, students experience both sides of the equation and add valuable sensory input inside their mind. An Asperger syndrome child often finds it difficult to cope with the social proximity and he stands very far or too close during a conversation with his partner. He also is not conscious about the exact distance in the space and face difficulties in justifying the exact distance between certain objects. But Aikido can teach him these techniques at ease. When throwing his opponent, a child must control his own movement in space in order to be in a position to throw his opponent. Conversely, when in the opposite role, students roll either forward or backward that provides vestibular stimulation as well as tactile contact with the mat.

Aikido also teaches a child how to read cues and maintain proper body distance for conversation. Every technique done with a partner may be seen as a physical representation of a certain kind of conversation. If the attacking partner is too far away, then you may not reach to grab him. If he is too close then he may be vulnerable to an offensive strike by the partner. These physical activities put precise information inside the mind of Asperger child and he learns how to control his motor skills and movements naturally.

5 Tips for Parents of Child Suffering from Asperger Syndrome

If you want your child to live a normal and happy life, then follow these simple tips: --

Teach your child some practical skills so that he integrates into social settings. The child may benefit from practicing appropriate openers like "Can you help me with this?"

Encourage your child to look at what other children of his age are doing. Many children suffering from Asperger syndrome reported that they have learned social skills through watching and emulating what others do in certain situations.

Teach the importance of eye contact to your child. Children suffering from Asperger syndrome often find it difficult to maintain an eye contact with others during a conversation.

Discuss about a personal feeling and thought the child experienced during his school sessions. It can be helpful to talk about how he or she feels in various circumstances that he met with during his or her school sessions and his feeling about it.

Praise your child in natural occurring situations when he or she uses appropriate skills. For example you can comment that "You were being very helpful to your siblings."

Chapter 3: Characteristics Of Asperger Syndrome

Each and every person is intrinsically different, especially when they have been diagnosed with Asperger Syndrome. An individual might have all or only some of the described behaviors to have a diagnosis of AS. These behaviors are first identified when a person is experiencing extreme difficulty in developing age-appropriate peer relationships. Children with AS are often more comfortable with adults than with other children. Once this behavior is noticed, other behaviors come to light including changes in eye gaze, facial expressions, body posture, and gestures that regulate social interaction.

With continuous observation, more questionable behaviors can be noticed.

These include inflexible adherence to routine perseveration, fascination with maps, globes, and routes, difficulty judging personal space, sensitivity to the environment, loud noises, clothing, food textures and odors. When interacting with other people, a person with Asperger Syndrome will have a challenge understanding the other person's feelings, and is likely to have socially and emotionally inappropriate responses.

Knowing and understanding the actions that have been described, helps one achieve the motivation of wanting to survive with their loved ones who have been diagnosed. Even though it may not be easy to detect these behaviors, with loving concern and interaction, one has the ability to notice changes in personality.

The person with Asperger's desires to fit in socially and have friends, but they have a great deal of difficulty making effective social connections. Many of them are at risk of developing mood disorders, such as anxiety or depression, especially in adolescence.

Understanding Communication from an Asperger Child

Under a range of circumstances, parents and guardians of children with AS often feel unable to communicate and interact with their child, basically because they are unsure of how to do so. What they need to relearn is how to communicate effectively in this situation.

Communication happens when one person sends a message to another person either verbally or non-verbally. Interaction happens when two people, for example, an adult and a child, respond to one another – resulting in two-way communication.

Most children with AS have difficulty interacting with others. This is because in order to be successful at interactions, the child needs to respond to others when they are approached by them or to be able to initiate interactions. Although many children with AS are able to do this when they want something, they tend not to use interaction to show people things or to be sociable.

It is important to remember that communication and interaction do not have to involve the use of language and speech. Many children with AS are delayed in their use of language and shy away from using speech. Therefore, other methods of communication need to be established before speech and language will follow.

The child may appear not to hear what is said to them, fail to respond to their name and/or be indifferent to any attempts of communication that are made. The use of everyday opportunities and play can encourage communication and interaction with a child that has AS.

The way in which the child communicates needs to be observed in order to further develop their communicative strengths and needs. For example, if the child is not using any sound or speech, rather than communicating with them through words, try using gesture. The child with AS may use some of the following characters to communicate with others: crying, taking the adults hand to the object they desire, looking at the object they desire, reaching, using pictures and echolalia.

Echolalia is the repetition of other people's words and is a common feature of the child with AS. Initially when the child uses echolalia it is likely that they are repeating words that they do not understand and are doing so with no communicative intent. However, echolalia is a good sign, as it shows that the child's communication is developing – in time, the child will begin to use the repeated words and phrases to communicate something significant. For example, the child may memorize the words that were said to them when they were asked if they would like a drink, and use them later in a different situation to ask a question of their own.

In understanding the purpose of the child's communication, you can help the child find more ways and more reasons to communicate.

You should consider these two types of communication:

Pre-intentional Communication: This is when the child says or does things without intending to affect those around them. This type of communication can be used by the child to calm and focus themselves, or as a reaction to an upsetting/fun experience.

Intentional Communication: This is when the child says or does things with the purpose of sending a message to another person. This type of communication can be used to protest about what they are being asked to do and to make requests.

Intentional communication is easier for the child once they have learned that their actions have an effect on other people – the move from pre-intentional communication to intentional communication is a big step for the child.

It is believed that it is helpful to view children with AS to being on a continuum in terms of their intentional communication. At one end of the continuum are children who communicate mainly to get the things they want, at the other end are children who communicate for many reasons, such as to ask questions, comment on something or to be sociable.

Stages of Communication

The stage of communication that the child has reached depends on three things:

Their ability to interact with another person.

How and why they communicate.

Their understanding.

Stage One – The Own Agenda Stage

A child at this stage of communication will appear uninterested in the people around them and will tend to play alone. Their communication will be mainly pre-intentional. The majority of children first diagnosed are at this stage.

Stage Two – The Requester Stage

At this stage the child has begun to realize that their actions have an effect on other people. They are likely to communicate to the adult their wants and what they enjoy by pulling them towards objects, areas, or games.

Stage Three – The Early Communicator Stage

At this stage the child's interactions will begin to increase in length and become more intentional. The child may also begin to echo some of the things that they hear to communicate their needs. Gradually the child will begin to point to things they want to show the adult and begin to shift their gaze. This is a sign that child is beginning to engage in a two-way interaction.

Stage Four – The Partner Stage

When the child reaches this stage they have become a more effective communicator. The child will be using speech to talk and will be able to carry out a simple conversation. While the child may appear confident and capable when using communication in familiar environments like at home, they may struggle when they enter unfamiliar territory like at a new nursery or school. It is in this situation that they may use memorized phrases and can often appear to be ignoring their communication partner by speaking over them and ignoring the rules of turn taking.

Chapter 4: "Asper -- What?"

Asperger Syndrome---it's not easy to pronounce; it's not easy to understand; and, it's not easy to accept that you or your loved one may be suffering from this condition. If there is one thing you need to know now, it's that, there is definitely reason to hope in spite of all the challenges that can be expected in dealing with Asperger Syndrome.

Tell-Tale signs

Just like many diseases, acceptance does not come easy for someone diagnosed with Asperger Syndrome (AS) and his family. AS, being a form of disability has an entire spool of stigma and stereotypes attached to it. It is the negative societal perceptions that often hinder a person with AS access to early diagnosis and prompt treatment.

The earlier a person with AS is properly diagnosed, the better his chances are of coping better with his condition. Early signs and symptoms of AS, when immediately recognized by his family or by a physician, particularly among small children, can make a huge difference in helping the patient and his loved ones cope more effectively with AS.

Listed below are behaviors that may indicate a child or an adult has AS. When and where you recognize any of the following, consult with your family physician immediately and request for diagnosis when necessary.

A person who has AS may:

•Have difficulty or trouble empathizing with others, and may even reach a point where they seem to not care about other peoples' feelings at all;

•Seem incapable of relating well with others or, even seem to be completely uninterested with people and any sort of social conversation or exchange;

•Have difficulty expressing their feelings or even showing any emotion at all;

•Be unable to direct his sight or gaze at a person talking to him or, at an object a person is pointing at;

•Appears to keep to himself, likes being alone, and avoids eye contact as much as possible;

•Have a strong tendency to repeat words or actions over and over but not really able to communicate effectively what he means to say or to accomplish whatever he means to do;

- Appear to be distracted, disturbed, and confused, even perplexed and mad when changes are introduced in his routine;

- On the contrary, he may seem to be overly focused and fixated on people and objects but still, remains clueless as to how to approach and interact with people and things; and,

- Have unexpected or strange reactions to stimuli, like the way things smell or look or feel.

These are but a few of the tell-tale signs that a person may have AS. Your physician will be in a better position to make a correct and reliable diagnosis. Still, the diagnosis begins at home. As soon as you recognize and accept that something could be wrong with your loved one, it's time you took personal initiative to seek professional help.

What is Asperger Syndrome?

You ask, what exactly is Asperger Syndrome? AS is a developmental disability that impairs an affected person's ability to relate with others and behave according to societal norms, that includes limitations mostly in social and communication skills. AS-affected individuals have a different way of sifting knowledge and learning from experiences. In fact, people diagnosed with AS have been observed to be either severely challenged or extremely intelligent.

AS is just one of the neurodevelopmental disorders in the full range of what is known as Autism Spectrum Disorder (ASD). Other disorders considered as ASD include pervasive developmental disorder not otherwise specified (PDD-NOS), childhood disintegrative disorder, and autistic disorder. These conditions share similar signs and symptoms as that of AS but, with AS being considered to be the mildest form of ASD.

AS was first recognized and diagnosed in 1944 by Austrian pediatrician, Hans Asperger. However, AS did not receive medical recognition as a health condition until the 1990s, when the World Health Organization listed AS in the 1992 International Classification of Diseases. In mid-2013, due to the lack of scientific basis to make a distinction between AS and ASD, AS was lumped with ASD.

Does he or doesn't he?

People with AS are born with it or, have developed these in early childhood. There is only one way to know for sure: a medical diagnosis is called for to ascertain that an individual does have AS.

Ideally, people with AS should be diagnosed as early as they turn two years old so that treatment options can immediately begin to be explored for them to maximize benefits. However, because AS is a developmental anomaly, and children's developmental progress are just starting to show around their early years, it's easy to shrug off AS to be merely an acceptable delay. It becomes more difficult when parents and other adults around the affected child struggle to accept that something could be wrong, even when the signs are stark and evident.

Formal diagnosis of AS happens when the child's pediatrician observes developmental gaps during a regular medical checkup. Once the attending physician suspects something could be wrong, a series of assessments follows which calls for the expertise of other specialists that may include a psychiatrist, psychologist, and neurologist who, together as a team, evaluate the mental, psychological, speech, and psychomotor wellness of the patient.

A standard procedural diagnosis of AS, however, has yet to be established. As such, the evaluation process can be very fluid and highly subjective which makes misdiagnosis extremely likely, because what may appear to be AS for a specialist may be perfectly normal for another.

The Reality of Asperger Syndrome

"Your child has AS," your physician says. What do you do? What does that mean to your child and to you?

Why s/he? Why you?

It's likely you'll question why, of all people, you and your loved one have been chosen to cope with AS. You might even start blaming yourself for this "unfortunate" circumstance---if only you hadn't, if only you did so and so then, perhaps, your child wouldn't have AS.

There may be many different factors that make a child more likely to have an ASD, including environmental, biologic and genetic factors. It is possible that these factors may put some people at higher risk for ASD. However, since many of these alleged risk factors are beyond your control, what that simply means is that there's nothing you could have done to make the situation any different.

It's easy to feel alone, isolated, and peculiarly different when you have AS or, need to cope with AS for the love of a loved one. It may make you feel better to know that other people are going through the same challenges, many of whom have been very successful in coping with AS.

While there are no statistics that specifically paint a picture of the current AS situation, according to the US Center for Disease Control and Prevention, one in 68 births developed ASD in 2010, as compared to only one in 150 births in 2000—over 119 per cent increase in prevalence. Globally, an estimated one per cent of the world's population has ASD.

Can AS ever be overcome?

There is no available cure for AS, neither can AS ever be overcome. When it comes to AS, early diagnosis and early introduction of interventions are key requirements in raising an independent, AS-challenged adult. Depending on the support obtained by an Aspie (that is, an AS-challenged individual), most especially from family members, he will need more or need less help going through daily tasks and chores as he grows up.

A typical therapy program for an Aspie will consist of several components, each addressing the unique limitations and capabilities of each patient. The most appropriate and successful programs are those which are not only tailored to an Aspie's personality but also take into consideration the patient's interests.

Listed below are some of the most common challenges Aspies are faced with, along with the corresponding activities incorporated in their therapy program to address the problem:

• Poor social skills. Talk to a therapist who specializes in AS and autism in general. Ask his other patients about improvements in their condition or, speak to their parents or guardians in the case of children. Make sure you know the nitty-gritties of the program being prescribed to your AS-challenged loved one, and that the strategies being employed have been proven to deliver positive improvements.

Aspies, their families, and their friends can help improve an Aspie's social skills simply by paying attention to his interests. Take time to develop the same interests or find somebody who shares the same interests as he does and encourage your affected loved one to interact with this person on a regular basis.

- Difficulty processing and showing appropriate emotions and behavior towards others and specific situations. Aspies can become easily agitated by mere changes in their routines because that violates their expectations.

While a typical individual readily picks up socially appropriate manners and behaviors just by experience and observation, an Aspie experiences difficulties processing emotions and controlling their behavior to conform with social norms. That can be traced back to some delayed developments or irregularities happening in their brain. This also explains the close links between AS and associated mental health conditions that include anxiety and depression.

Aspies tend to use their intellect more, and use their emotions less. They are almost always behind their counterparts when it comes to emotional maturity. It will help to talk an Aspie through a situation and the specific emotions he is feeling. The situation and the emotions need to be broken down into smaller bits of information to simplify them and, more importantly, to help an Aspie process each segment clearly, carefully, and maturely.

If you don't feel confident you can give this to your loved one who is an Aspie, seek professional help but first, try to get your loved one to agree to talk to a professional because matters that involve emotions tend to be very personal.

- Slow progress in speech and motor skills. In general, Aspies vary greatly in skill sets where they excel and where they lag behind. It is important for loved ones to pay closer attention so that areas where an Aspie is slow or weak may be addressed, and for areas where they excel to be harnessed.

Speech and motor skills trainings are a typical component of any therapy program designed for Aspies. Some may need continued coaching well into their adult years.

There are many ways for an Aspie or his loved ones to help improve his condition.

Whichever area needs addressing, the starting points remain the same: paying close attention, recognizing a possible concern, and seeking help. Diagnosing his needs, possible solutions, and continued progress monitoring must be done in partnership (stress on "in partnership") with a qualified professional.

It is never acceptable to pass on the responsibility of supporting a loved one with Aspie to a hired caregiver. If you are serious that you would like to see improvements in your loved one's progress, you must become involved in his situation, and that includes making sure he is getting the appropriate therapy program. Family members must receive continuous counseling as well to help them better deal better and better support a member who has Aspie.

Always treat your Aspie-challenged loved one with respect. Take his limitations seriously; most especially when you see signs of associated mental health conditions like anxiety, isolation, and depression seriously. Always seek professional help. Never shrug off any potentially problematic behaviors as just a normal part of dealing with AS. Ask when you don't understand, and keep searching for answers and opportunities for your loved one's improvement.

Hang in there. AS may never be overcome but, you and your family, with much love and genuine care for each other, will overcome the challenges of AS together.

Chapter 5: Overview Of The Asperger Syndrome

It is unfortunate that children sometimes show signs and symptoms which have been attributed to neurodevelopmental disorders. These disorders have to do with social deficits, difficulties in communication, repetitive behaviors, intensely focused interests, issues in sensory perception, and sometimes delays in cognitive functions.

Before 2013, all of the above were classified as **autism**. After careful studies, it was discovered that four different and distinct disorders existed, and therefore, what was previously known and defined as **autism**, would hence forth be named **autism spectrum** or **autistic spectrum of disorders.** The differences lie mostly in the symptoms exhibited in each case. The four distinct disorders are:

A) Pervasive developmental disorder not otherwise specified (PDD-NOS).

The condition is diagnosed whenever the symptoms exhibited do not match the criteria defined in any of the other three categories. This classification is also one of the five pervasive developmental disorders that are not necessarily associated with any form of autism.

To receive a diagnosis, it is necessary for a team of specialists to be involved in the process and that an individual suspected of displaying PDD-NOS undergoes a full set of diagnostic evaluations, including:

Thorough examination of the historical record in social, adaptive, and motor skills, as well as communication and medical issues.

Scores on behavioral rating scales.

Observations of current behavioral patterns.

Psychological evaluation.

Educational evaluation.

Evaluation of the current communication skills.

Evaluating of the current occupation.

Researchers face a methodology problem with PDD-NOS, as the group of people who are diagnosed is heterogeneous and there is but only a brief case definition of PDD-NOS as a "sub-threshold" category.

It would appear from the clinical evidence that there are fewer intellectual deficits involved for children with PDD-NOS than in classical autism. Additionally, it is possible for these children to be submitted for evaluation at a later age than with the other three disorders of the autism spectrum.

B) Childhood disintegrative disorder

The condition is also known as the **Heller's Syndrome** or **disintegrative psychosis**. The characteristics defining this disorder are delays in the development of age-relevant language, poor social interactions and weak motor skills. This was actually the first form of autism to be discovered in 1908, and it is also the rarest. Theodor Heller, who initially described it (and consequently gave his name), called it **dementia infantilis.**

Perhaps the most crucial characteristic of this condition is that it is not made apparent immediately. In the majority of cases, there is a period of normal development for the child before the problems begin to appear. In some cases, this regression is so dramatic that the child is not even aware of it and will never ask about what is happening to him or her.

Most of the time, it is diagnosed when previously attained skills have been lost. It can happen any time during the normal development of a child, but typically onset is around the age of three. The skills that may be lost are included in at least two of the following six areas of developmental functionalities:

The ability to produce speech coherent enough to communicate a message. This is also known as **expressive language**.

The ability to listen to others and understand the message that is communicated. Also known as **receptive language.**

Skills that pertain to social and self-care issues.

Control of the bladder and bowel movements.

The ability of imaginative play.

Motor skills.

For these six classifications, the once-acquired skills have been almost completely lost between the ages of 2 and 10. But in order for the diagnosis to be CDD, there must also be impairment or complete absence in at least two of the following areas:

Social interaction

Communication

Patterns of restrictive and repetitive behavior and / or interests

CDD is also a disorder classification of which some of the underlying causes have been identified. (It has been linked with lipid storage diseases, subacute sclerosing panencephalitis and tuberous sclerosis.) These findings have raised considerable debates and controversies in reference to the right methods of treatment.

C) Classical Autism

If a child begins to display, within the first years of his or her life, symptoms of impaired social interaction, difficulties in verbal and non-verbal communication and behavioral patterns that are restricted and repetitive, it is most probable that the diagnosis will be standard autism.

This disorder is attributed to genetic and environmental issues, along with the use of agents that may cause birth defects. It is highly heritable, and for a successful diagnosis, the prerequisite is that the symptoms appear before the age of three.

Unlike with Asperger Syndrome, after the onset of autism there are only a small number of patients that can take care of themselves without supervision once they have reached adulthood.

A worrisome statistic is that the percentage of the appearance of autism within the general population has increased dramatically since the 1980s and the standardization of diagnostic tests. As of 2010, it was estimated that 1 or 2 individuals out of every 1,000 people on a worldwide basis suffer from classical autism. While it is not sex discriminant, the frequency of onset is five times greater in boys than in girls.

D)
Asperger Syndrome

The condition is characterized by the presence of all the symptoms that appear in the autism spectrum of disorders:

Difficulty in social functionality and interaction

Difficulty in verbal and non-verbal communication

Patterns of restricted and repetitive behavior

Restrictive and repetitive interests

Physical clumsiness

Atypical use of language

The last two symptoms are not required for the diagnosis of the syndrome, but they are present very frequently among the patients.

The discussion in this book will focus on Asperger Syndrome, its characteristics, classification, and all of the pertinent details which will allow for a better understanding. In addition, the accumulation of knowledge about the circumstances and reference information will help clarify what it is and what can be done about it.

Causes

Science and research have not yet defined what exactly it is that causes the syndrome. Part of the hypothesis formed thus far includes genetic factors, but a certain genetic cause or gene has yet to be identified. Nor was brain imaging successful in defining a common pathology, and there is only very limited and sketchy information on the effects of particular interventions.

Furthermore, there is no single treatment that can address all the symptoms and work on all patients. Currently the sets of remedies explored have focused on behavioral therapy that addresses the specific inadequacies and deficits presented on a case-by-case basis.

Returning to the genetic hypothesis of Asperger's, this is supported by the observations of a phenotypic variability that has been seen in children suffering from AS. For the uninitiated, phenotypes are the composites of an organism's traits or observable characteristics. These include morphology, biochemical properties, physiological properties, as well as the organism's behavior and its products (the nest of a bird is a product of the bird's behavior, for example).

Further evidence is provided by the fact that the syndrome tends to run in families and that the genetic component in this syndrome appears to be stronger than the genetic component found in the other disorders of the autistic spectrum.

It is also possible that siblings may display similar symptoms but at different intensities and that one member of the family may actually be diagnosable with AS, while the other members exhibit similar behaviors but in a much more limited form which is not actually diagnosable.

There is a working hypothesis undergoing research that involves a common group of genes where the presence of some particular **alleles** may result in a greater vulnerability of an individual developing AS. Should this indeed be the case, it is the combination of the alleles involved that determines the severity of the disorder and the intensity of the symptoms exhibited.

For those not familiar with the biology, an **allele** is something like an isotope. Genes are not always exactly the same. They appear in a number of alternative forms. One of these alternative forms is called an allele. The best example of what an allele is may be the color of the skin. The difference between Asian, Caucasian, and African races in terms of the color of the skin is based on a different allele of the same gene.

The same stands true if the allele does not refer to a specific gene but a **gene locus,** which is actually the location within a gene, a chromosome or a DNA sequence in which an allele is found. It may even be that a specific DNA sequence that is found in a specific location is, itself, an allele.

For those who want to study the allele hypothesis further, they should first acquire further knowledge of the human genome and the genetic maps, as these are where determining the location of a specific biological trait is occurring.

Further scientific observations link Asperger's to exposure of the mother to teratogen agents within the first eight weeks of conception. Teratogens are the agents that cause birth defects. Some teratogens are:

A) Toxic substances **such as drugs**

Either for pharmaceutical or for recreational purposes, any medical compounds that act during the embryonic and fetal development may produce an alteration in a form or a function.

B) Environmental toxins

There is evidence that:

Polychlorinated biphenyls

Phthalates

Phenols

Organo-chlorine pesticides

Polybrominated diphenyl ethers

Perfluorinated compounds

Polycyclic aromatic hydrocarbons pose a significant danger to fetuses during their development stages.

C) Vertically transmitted infections

These are infections caused by bacteria, viruses or parasites. They are passed from the mother to the child during the embryonic and fetal stages of pregnancy or during childbirth.

D) Malnutrition

This is a condition in which the body is deprived of specific nutrients. For example, a condition called **spina bifida** is caused by the lack of folic acid in the dietary habits of the mother during pregnancy.

E)
Physical restraints

There is a condition called oligohydramnios. It describes the decrease of the volume of amniotic fluid which may be enough to significantly affect the morphogenesis of a fetus. This is an example of physical issues that may cause teratogenesis.

Exposure to these agents may explain why the disorder appears so early in childhood. Other causes examined pertain to environmental factors, but no theories are yet confirmed by research. On the contrary, some of them have been disproven and consequently dismissed.

The Mechanism

Asperger Syndrome, whatever the causes may be, seems to affect either the total or a major part of functional brain systems, instead of imposing a localized effect. Some researchers speculate that it may be necessary to separate the research for this specific disorder from the research conducted for the other disorders of the autistic spectrum, as they hypothesize that the mechanism is actually different here and it distinctively points to alterations in the brain development a short while after the embryo was conceived.

These alterations seem to be attributed to a migration of embryonic cells during the development of the fetus that is abnormal and affects the final structure of the brain and its connectivity. The theory supposes that there are high-level neural connections that are underperforming, which means that the synchronization between the functions, combined with the presence of excessive low-level processes, suffers greatly. This combination of factors is most likely the reason behind the delays in the cognitive functions and the loss of already attained skills.

The theory is supported by neuroanatomical studies, in association with the exposure to teratogens, which provide evidence that strongly support that the mechanism of alterations occurs in the development of the cerebellum right after the embryo's conception.

Other theories that have been developed and pertain to the mechanism behind Asperger's are the **weak central coherence theory**, which assumes that a limited ability to see the big picture is the cause behind the core disorder, and the **mirror neuron system theory,** which assumes that the alterations in the development stage interfere with the fundamental learning process of imitation and lead to the core feature of Asperger's, the impairment of social interaction.

Diagnosis

To find out if a child suffers from Asperger Syndrome, the standard criteria require the impairment of the social functions and interaction and the observance of stereotypic patterns of repetitive and restrictive behavior. This impairment should not extend to the language or other cognitive development. Furthermore, there has to be significant impairment in the everyday functioning of the child.

This usually happens between the ages of 4 and 11, and to make sure that the diagnosis is correct, the child should be assessed by a team of multidisciplinary observers that will render clinical judgment after the examination of three separate tests.

The examination should include:

Evaluation of the neurological condition

Evaluation of the genetics involved

Cognitive tests

Evaluation of the psychomotor functions

Evaluation of the strengths and weakness in verbal and nonverbal communication

Evaluation of the learning and knowledge acquisition style

The ability for independent living

The relevant interviews include:

The **Revised Autism Diagnostic Interview,** which is a semi-structured parent interview

The **Autism Diagnostic Observation Schedule,** which is a conversation with the child and an interview based on play.

It is of utmost importance that the diagnosis occurs as early as possible and that there is no misdiagnosis involved. This latter case especially may cause additional problems, should medication be prescribed that will actually worsen the behavioral patterns.

Another reason for the earliest possible diagnosis is the fact that diagnosing adults is much more difficult. All the tests have been designed to address children and the symptoms exhibited change as the individual grows up. A very painstaking and time-consuming procedure would be required to diagnose an adult.

It would need to subject the person to a thorough clinical examination, and it would include a complete medical history as accumulated by the individual himself or herself. Additionally, interviews should be conducted with people who are familiar to and have detailed knowledge of the person's history and who can attest to behavioral patterns and changes.

Diagnosing Asperger's gets even more complicated in both children and adults as a differential diagnosis may be required which would consider a great number of affiliated disorders such as:

Disorders of the schizophrenia spectrum

O.C.D. (obsessive-compulsive disorder)

Major depressive disorder

Semantic pragmatic disorder

Nonverbal learning disorder

Tourette syndrome

Stereotypic movement disorder

Bipolar disorder

Social and cognitive deficits that are produced by damage to the brain, including alcohol abuse

A major problem that has surfaced recently in reference to the diagnosis is that the cost involved and the difficulty of the screening process, along with the increasing popularity in using medication and the expansion of the benefits received, has produced an incentive to health providers to over-diagnose AS.

Screening

Before any child, adolescent or adult is put through the diagnosis process described above, they are put through a screening procedure which determines if any further testing is merited. This screening process begins with the parents.

They are typically able to identify even slight differences in the behavior of their child as early as the 30th month of age. It follows logically that they will require the opinion of a pediatrician or a general practitioner. They will determine, after a routine examination, if further investigation is needed. Should this be the case, a number of screening tools are available. These are:

The Asperger Syndrome Diagnostic Scale (ASDS)

The Childhood Autism Spectrum Test (CAST) (renamed from Childhood Asperger Syndrome Test)

The Autism Spectrum Screening Questionnaire (ASSQ)

The Krug Asperger's Disorder Index (KADI)

The Gilliam Asperger's Disorder Scale (GADS)

The Autism Spectrum Quotient (ASQ), which has different version for children, adolescents and adults

All of the above will indicate if there is an autism spectrum disorder but not which one. This is why the rest of the diagnostic process is necessary.

Prognosis

Twenty percent of people diagnosed with Asperger's in childhood may experience a lessening of the symptoms to the point that they no longer qualify as patients of the disorder when they reach adulthood. Another great percentage may experience a lessening of the symptoms, but will still be considered patients after the end of adolescence. In both cases, some social functions and communication skills may still be impaired.

There is no difference in the life expectancy of AS patients, but there is an increased chance that they will succumb to comorbid psychiatric conditions like depressive disorder and anxiety.

The most positive prognosis is that AS does not seem to affect the ability of some individuals to achieve, as amply displayed by the Nobel Prize awardee Vernon L. Smith.

The most critical aspect in the prognosis of Asperger Syndrome is the education of families and teachers. They can play the most significant role in helping their children (or students) and participate positively in the behavioral therapies. It is equally important that these people are able to cope with the situation, which may become extremely straining, especially the later the syndrome is diagnosed.

If the severity of the syndrome warrants such an action, it may be necessary to submit the children with AS to special educational facilities specially equipped and trained to handle their social and behavioral deficiencies.

Legal Implications

Another aspect to consider in Asperger's are the legal implications. Patients of the disorder may become subjects of exploitation by other individuals, or they may not be aware of the implications involved in their social actions. This is a concept that has caused much debate.

The aspies themselves (at least those with sufficient levels of cognitive abilities) do not consider Asperger's as a disorder but as a genetic difference, similar to homosexuality. If this notion prevails, then the aspies must be held responsible for all of their actions, regardless of their condition, in a court of law.

On the other hand, if the medical opinion prevails, aspies may stand to receive judgments of diminished capacity, when it comes to their actions, regardless of whether their condition allows them to have complete awareness of the consequences of what they have done.

In any case, Asperger Syndrome needs a lot more scientific studies and research that will provide a unified and definite answer as to the causes, the context and what must be done in order to satisfactorily remedy the situation. The aspies themselves may choose to reject this remedy if they are judged capable enough to decide for themselves, but the option must be available for those who choose not to suffer from society's misgivings, misconceptions and misunderstandings, or to be treated like curses or abominations.

Chapter 6: Aspergers Syndrome Treatments, Therapies And Medication.

There is not one set remedy for Asperger's syndrome. You will not find a medication that will cure a child with Aspergers. Instead, you will find several treatments to help with the problems connected with Asperger's syndrome. Here we will examine a few of the treatments employed with Asperger's syndrome.

Social skills training

Kids with Asperger's syndrome have a hard time understanding facial gestures, and tone of voice. They tend to take everything said to them very literally. They do not know when a person is joking with them. Children can be coached to recognize changes in people's voice, and what different facial gestures mean. They, in addition, need to be instructed on how to use better eye contact. This type of training can help their child to make friends. They're taught how to act around other people. Some children with Aspergers want to be around other kids, they just are unaware of how to act with them. They can be coached how to act when out shopping, or at a restaurant.

Cognitive behavior therapy

This type of therapy instructs the youngster with Asperger's syndrome to find ways to cope. They are taught ways to slim down anxiety. They learn how to spot a predicament that can result in them trouble. Then they learn methods to cope when they're in that position. Aspergers children often have a great deal of anxiety. They have a difficult time in social settings.

They can have panic attacks or complete meltdowns. Cognitive therapy teaches them ways to stop the meltdowns from occurring. This therapy will teach a youngster with Aspergers that when they feel an unwanted behavior coming near something they are able to do to stop it.

They're taught how to remove themselves from a predicament that ensures they are uneasy.

Medicine

There is no medication that will treat Aspergers. Nonetheless, there is medicine to help with a few of the symptoms of Aspergers. Many kids with Aspergers have anxiety and depression. There are treatments that can assist relieve these problems. Relieving the anxiety can help their child feel more leisurely in social settings. Drugs like these can have side effects. You will have to monitor your child's behavior while they are on the medication. Some children with Aspergers have a hard time sleeping. There are medicines to help youngster sleep.

Being a parent education

There is training for the mothers and fathers of Asperger's children. This training incorporates ways you can handle behaviors. Learning things that can assist to calm your child down when they are having a meltdown, or anxiety attack. Mothers and fathers are taught ways of using reward systems to control behavior problems. They are taught how to manage the behaviors in the house. This helps them to deal with behaviors away too.

With these treatments, the life of an Asperger's child can be easier. If no therapy is given kids with Aspergers can have trouble with depression, and anxiety. They have such a difficult time coping with people socially they could go to alcohol or drugs to unwind them. Getting a therapy plan that works is a principal priority for your Aspergers child.

COGNITIVE BEHAVIORAL THERAPY (CBT) AND ASPERGER SYNDROME

Asperger Syndrome cannot be cured. However, a mixture of treatments makes it possible for those diagnosed with this form of autism to manage the symptoms that negatively affect their daily life.

Most children and adults with this condition go on to lead fulfilling lives with a personalized mixture of therapy and (sometimes) medication.

One of the most popular methods for dealing with Asperger Syndrome is Cognitive Behavioral Therapy.

About CBT

Cognitive Behavioral Therapy (CBT) is goal-oriented and proactive, where the therapist and patient work together to find a strategy for handling specific problems. This is different from regular talk-based therapy in that it goes beyond psychological assessment to hammering out particular patterns of distress, maladaptive thinking, and so forth, and working on ways to solve them. Developing coping mechanisms, positive thinking, and effective behaviors are such solutions.

How it can help?

CBT can help those with Asperger Syndrome manage their obsessive interests and reliance on routines; it's also useful in developing methods for improving social interaction. It does this by having the patient identify the anxiety that comes with relying on routines-or, in the case of socialization, what parts of conversation and relationships confuse them. After these problems are identified, the therapist and patient work together to create exercises and step-by-step instructions for reducing anxiety and knowing what to do in social situations.

Because it demands the patient to get in touch with his or her feelings and work through negative emotions, CBT has also proven to be effective in treating the depression and anxiety disorders that often accompany Asperger Syndrome.

Difficulties

Although generally very useful, those with an Autism Spectrum Disorder may have a particularly difficult time with CBT. Most patients only go once or twice a week for an hour at a time for a set duration. Other patients may have to go more often or for longer because it is more difficult for them to communicate and identify emotions.

But this should not be a point of discouragement. Despite occasional setbacks and slower progress, CBT helps those with Asperger Syndrome with their lives in general. It is a holistic treatment that targets many symptoms at once, unlike many medications and other forms of therapy.

CBT is a vital part of living with Asperger Syndrome and other forms of autism. It can help reduce reliance on medication and improve the overall happiness of those with Asperger Syndrome-two huge achievements. But most importantly, the exercises and coping mechanisms learned in CBT are indispensable tools that can be used every day.

TREATMENT FOR ASPERGER SYNDROME

Asperger syndrome is a neurobiological condition that affects children and adults. Many people feel it is a form of high functioning autism and it falls in the group of conditions of spectrum disorder or pervasive personality disorder. It affects the ability of the person to socialize and communicate effectively with others. Individuals often exhibit social communication, social interaction, and social imagination.

At this time doctors and researchers have not found a cause or cure for Asperger syndrome. There has been some research to indicate that individuals who suffer from this condition have had permanent changes to their frontal lobe. These changes make a difference in the ability of the brain to process social activities.

In 1944 Hans Asperger labeled this disorder autistic psychopathy and published a paper describing the symptoms and behaviors. However, it wasn't until 1994 that the disability was recognized in the DSM-IV. Throughout those years, and the many different research studies which have been performed, the exact cause of this disorder has never been found.

While there is currently no cure for Asperger syndrome there are treatment protocols that help both adults and children to learn how to interact more successfully in social situations.

Treatment which may be recommended will depend upon the individual's level of adaptive functioning. Just as with autism, there is a range of disability or functionality of individuals who have Asperger's.

Resources that are available for children and adults with Asperger syndrome are communication and social skills training which help individuals to learn the unwritten rules of socialization and communication. These are often too difficult for children in much the same way that students learn to speak a foreign language. This is because for children and adults with Asperger syndrome learning these social communication skills is a foreign language.

It is possible for children with Asperger syndrome to learn how to speak using a more natural rhythm as well as how to interpret communication such as gestures, eye contact, tone of voice, humor and sarcasm which usually fly right over the top of their heads.

Another behavioral therapy that may be recommended is cognitive behavior therapy. This technique is aimed at its decreasing problem behaviors such as interrupting, obsessions and angry outbursts. They also focused on helping children and adults to recognize a troubled situation, such as a new place or events, and then be able to select a specific strategy to cope.

While there is no medication specifically aimed at treatment of Asperger syndrome there are some symptoms that can be controlled, such as anxiety, depression or hyperactivity using medications. Most commonly, selective serotonin reuptake inhibitors, antipsychotics, and some stimulants are used to treat these problems.

Treatment outlook for individuals with Asperger syndrome is usually heavily correlated with the measured IQ. Those who have a high IQ will fare better and show greater improvements in social function than those who have a below average IQ.

Children who experience the symptoms of Asperger syndrome will also require a bit of assistance in the school system.

Schools that have a communications specialist with an interest in social skills training, opportunities for social interaction and structured settings, a concern for teaching real-life skills and a willingness to individualize the curriculum are best suited to help individuals who have Asperger syndrome. Parents should stay informed of what is happening in the child's classroom and maintain frequent communication with the teacher.

Even though a specific pill is not available for treatment for Asperger syndrome, and there is no cure, individuals who have this condition have a degree of adaptability to the environment when they are taught coping strategies and have a good support system in their relationships.

TREATMENT AVAILABLE FOR A CHILD WITH ASPERGER SYNDROME

Since a child with Asperger Syndrome shows patterns of behaviors and problems that differ widely from others, any typical treatment regimen or medication cannot be prescribed. However, there are several treatments that are proven to help a lot with the child's condition and his development. These include the following:

Parents Education And Training. The parents, aside from being the first teachers are the primary guardians who can reinforce help to a child with Aspergers. It is crucial that they're educated properly with the nature of the kid's condition. Therefore, as a child's parent, you should undergo this type of training so you can even teach your child with Asperger self-help abilities. Learning these skills helps children achieve maximum independence.

Social Skills Training. Since a child with Aspergers is having difficulty interacting with other individuals, even with kids of his age, the child must undergo social skills training. As a child's parent, you could start this training by yourself; however, it's more advantageous on your part and your child if you ask for the guidance of an expert. Specialized training programs exist for the development of social skills intended for children with Aspergers.

Language Development Programs. Even holding a normal conversation might be difficult for a child with Aspergers. While most individuals learn these skills by observing others, the people with Asperger's Syndrome might need personal coaching using specialized language development programs. For faster development, parents should contribute by teaching the kid to start a conversation in the most approachable manner. Body language and eye-contact are effective approaches which promote the connection between the parent and the kid.

Cognitive Behavioral Therapy. Psychological conditions such as Aspergers Syndrome in all ages might be treated utilizing this therapy.

This therapy applies approaches designed to modify the way a child thinks, feels and reacts to a situation. It targets the overall behavior of the child, especially the repetitive actions the child often does. A therapist has the capability to establish a connection between him and the child in a way that the child can feel comfortable and conditioned.

Tender Loving Care. Adults, especially the parents, play a significant role in the development of the kid with Aspergers by showing extensive care and love to this kid. Teachers, babysitters, the rest of the family members, close friends, and everyone else must get involved in the training and should sustain strong affection to the child for its faster development. Never let the child feel isolated to its environment. Instead, make the kid feel that it belongs wherever it gets involved with, especially at home and school. And in every action you make, do it with tender loving care.

HOW IS ASPERGER'S SYNDROME DIAGNOSED?

If you suspect your child to have this condition, bringing him or her to a doctor is a good idea. The doctor will ask you a series of questions regarding your child's behavior. Your child will undergo a series of tests analyzing his ability to communicate, express, read and write. Intellectual, emotional and psychological evaluations may be done as well. The evaluation might be made by a number of doctors since Asperger's is a bit hard to diagnose. Some may even mistake it for other developmental problems such as attention deficit/hyperactivity disorder or ADHD.

HOW IS ASPERGER'S SYNDROME TREATED?

As mentioned earlier, there is no exact cure for Asperger's. The doctors will only recommend medications and therapies to lessen their severity and help the child cope and live to his optimum potential. There are no exact medications for Asperger's, but the doctor can prescribe drugs to relieve depression, anxiousness, and agitation which the child can manifest anytime. Therapies are also advised to improve the child's ability to communicate and understand people, and to improve his social skills. They are taught the right way of expressing how they feel and how to understand nonverbal cues such as eye contact, facial expressions, and other gestures. The child is also taught of ways to cope with certain situations such as going to school, meeting other people or transferring to another location.

HOW CAN A PARENT HELP THE CHILD COPE?

Parents have the most important role in helping the child cope with this condition. They are the ones who have been with the child and are well-oriented about the situation.

You can learn about Asperger's. Education and information are very important in order to understand what your child is going through. You can ask your doctor, read medical books or journals, and research over the internet about the condition of your child. You can also read ways on how to cope with your child, especially during hard times.

Be familiar with your child's behavior. Not all children with Asperger's manifest the same symptoms and characteristics. By being familiar with your child's behavior, you also learn how to deal with it. Just have patience in going through tough times and show your child how supportive you can be.

Be active in therapies. Your child will undergo therapies until he or she is able to adjust. Be present in therapies so you can learn more about your child and his or her condition. Talk to the professionals in charge of the sessions so that you can also become part of the team.

Inform people about your child's condition. Some parents may be hesitant about telling people about their child, but it is important to let others know about it. Inform the school, teachers, and people in your neighborhood about your child's condition so they can also adjust to your child.

Since children with Asperger's may have awkward social skills, others may misinterpret this and be judgmental if they are not properly informed.

ALTERNATIVE THERAPIES AND TREATMENTS FOR ASPERGER

HERBS AND NATURAL REMEDIES

If you have a child that has been diagnosed with Asperger's syndrome, you want to find the best treatments available.

Aspergers cannot be cured however, because it is not a disease. Treatments for children with Aspergers are designed to help them function better in the areas the condition have affected them. Others have found the following treatments for Aspergers to be effective.

In a lot of instances, children affected by Aspergers require several different strategies and healing methods. While the accurate reason that Aspergers happens is a mystery, it does have an effect on how a person's brain works. For this reason, signals can from time to time be assisted from biofeedback. There are some inventive programs that imply some potential, which inform individuals with Aspergers how to change their brainwaves to assist in overcoming a variety of dilemmas.

While this kind of treatment for Aspergers is considered experimental and is not widely accepted, some researchers claim that it can be highly effective. Asperger's is not a disease and it's important that you and your child realize this and that it simply means a person's brain works differently. Evidence is starting to show that historic people such as Albert Einstein, Thomas Jefferson, Beethoven, and Mozart had Asperger's syndrome. By focusing on their strengths, people with this condition can do well in today's technological society. Of course, children with Aspergers do have challenges, and some face serious problems, but the point is to keep in mind that they can still be highly successful as well.

Some herbs and other natural remedies have been found to help treat Aspergers, as well. It is possible to use herbal remedies to help calm a child with

Aspergers down, help them focus, and to help reduce their anxiety.

For symptoms ranging from anxiety to depression, the supplement St. John's Wort can be used for both adults and children.

Passiflora also called passion flower, and chamomile is other herbal remedies that can be soothing to the nervous system. A homeopathic or herbal practitioner can give you more information on herbal remedies for treating specific symptoms of Aspergers.

Remember you are not alone as you face all the challenges that come with parenting a child with Aspergers. This condition is quite common, and fortunately, while there's no known cure, there are many ways to effectively deal with it. Some of the treatments discussed above may be of help to you and your family and make it a little easier to understand Asperger's syndrome.

USING HERBS AND NATURAL PRODUCTS TO TREAT ASPERGERS

When it comes to medicating children afflicted with Asperger's syndrome, you will probably need to be both tolerant and inventive, as all children are a bit different and you might need to try a variety of strategies prior to recognizing the ones that work optimally. While you should meet with a qualified physician, psychologists, and school administrators, bear in mind that you know your child better than anyone else, therefore you should also put your acumen and talent for cognizance to use. The following are some remedies for Aspergers that may work excellently for your child.

Changes to routine are especially hard for children with Aspergers to handle, therefore stability is very important. Assigning times for even simple tasks like free time, homework and mealtime will help give them structure in their routine. When choosing parenting styles many parents prefer to give their children more freedom, while others prefer this more rigid style. No matter what your preference is when it comes to kids with Aspergers, you aren't doing them a favor by giving them too much flexibility in such areas, as it will only confuse them.

Conclusion

Thank you again for downloading this book!

I hope this book was able to help you gain a more thorough understanding of Asperger's. You are doing a service to this world by expressing enough interest to invest in a more well-rounded perspective of a beautiful and often misunderstood condition. As small as this investment may seem at first, it stretches only as far as you are willing.

The next step is to use the information from this book to support loved ones and spread the message so that Asperger's can be more accurately represented and empathized with.

Thank you and good luck!

www.ingramcontent.com/pod-product-compliance
Lightning Source LLC
LaVergne TN
LVHW011951070526
838202LV00054B/4894